Smart Hygiene Solutions
Examples of Hygiene Methods & Tools and Tips

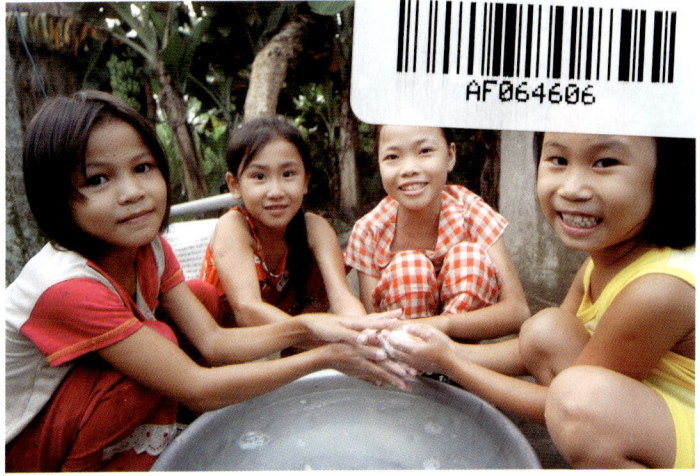

(Source: PLAN)

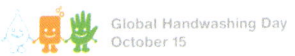

Global Handwashing Day
October 15

The first edition of this booklet was launched during the Global Handwashing Day Campaign 2010. Each year in October, Global Handwashing Day is the centerpiece of a week of activities that mobilise millions of people in more than 80 countries across all five continents to wash their hands with soap.
This booklet is the result of a successful cooperation between the Netherlands Water Partnership (NWP), Unilever, Aqua for All, PLAN Nederland, IRC International Water and Sanitation Centre and all other organizations indicated under Collaboration and Acknowledgement.

2 COLLABORATION

This publication is the result of a collaborative effort by a number of organisations:

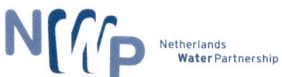

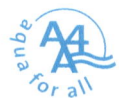

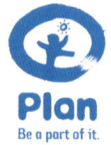

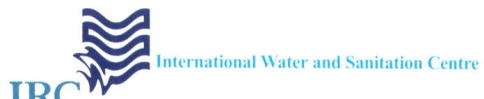

ACKNOWLEDGEMENT

We would like to thank the following organisations for their enthusiastic contribution to this booklet:

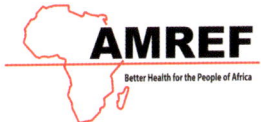
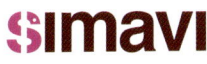
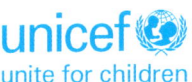
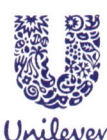

Coordination/ main writers: Plan Nederland: Sharon Roose, Aqua for All: Elbrich Spijksma,
IRC: Tettje van Daalen, NWP: Mascha Singeling
Editing   : Kathleen Shordt
Graphic Design   : Grafisch ontwerpbureau Agaatsz bNO, Meppel
Financial Support   : Unilever, Simavi, PLAN Nederland, Partners voor Water
Photos   : PLAN International, IRC, Aqua for All, Unicef
Printing   : High Trade, Zwolle

© 2010 KIT Publishers - Amsterdam
Kit Publishers
Mauritskade 63
PO Box 95001
1090 HA Amsterdam
W: www.kitpublishers.nl
E: publishers@kit.nl
ISBN 978 94 6022 127 9

TABLE OF CONTENT

FORWARD	5
SMART HYGIENE SOLUTIONS BOOKLET	7
WHAT IS HYGIENE?	8
WHAT IS HYGIENE PROMOTION?	12
METHODS OF HYGIENE PROMOTION	17
PARTICIPATORY STRATEGIES	18
SOCIAL MARKETING	22
TOTAL SANITATION	24
CLUBS	28
TOOLS ANDS TIPS FOR HYGIENE IMPROVEMENT	32
HAND WASHING	34
SAFE EXCRETA DISPOSAL	36
CLEAN WATER: TREATMENT, SAFE STORAGE AND ATTRACTION	38
MENSTRUAL HYGIENE	40
FOOD PREPARATION & STORAGE	42
VECTOR CONTROL	44
LITERATURE	51

FOREWORD

Approximately 120 million children are born in the developing world each year. Halve of these children will live in households without access to improved water and sanitation, which puts their survival and development at grave risk. As a result of poor hygiene and lack of access to water and sanitation, 1.5 million under five children die every year because of diarrhoeal diseases alone. Vast improvement in water, sanitation and hygiene are needed to meeting Millennium Development Goal Four- reducing death among children under the age of five by two-thirds by 2015.

The importance of hygiene in water and sanitation programmes has often been neglected. Too often improvement in hygiene was thought to follow automatically once water and sanitation facilities are in place. But in practice improving hygiene behaviour requires special attention.

Hand washing with soap is the most effective and inexpensive way to prevent diarrhoeal and acute respiratory infections, which take the lives of millions of children in developing countries every year. Yet, despite its lifesaving potential, hand washing with soap is seldomly practiced and difficult to promote.

To achieve behaviour change at the scale that's required to meet Millennium Development Goal 4, public and private sector organisations need to join forces, bringing their expertise and resources to the table to create campaigns that reach homes, schools and communities worldwide.

This is why Unilever through its lifebuoy brand has made the commitment to change the hand washing behaviour of one billion people by 2015. Together with a wide array of governments, international institutions, civil society organisations, NGOs, private companies and individuals around the globe, Unilever works to deliver a positive impact to everyday health through the hand washing campaign of its Lifebuoy product.

This booklet on Smart Hygiene Solutions, gives examples of approaches, tools and tips that aim to improve hygiene behaviour and environmental conditions. I hope this booklet helps to develop interventions that lead to sustainable changes in hygiene and contributes to the further improvement of everyday health in developing countries.

Dr Myriam Sidibe

Global Social Mission Manager for Lifebuoy
Unilever United Kingdom

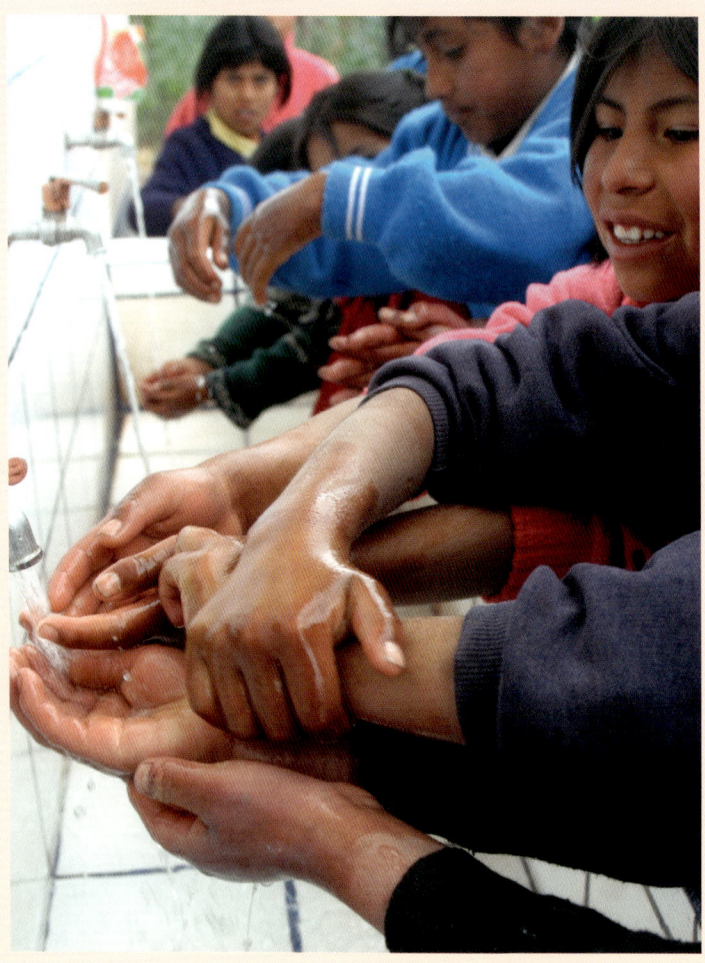
(Source: PLAN)

SMART HYGIENE SOLUTIONS BOOKLET

The Smart Hygiene Solutions booklet is written for non-governmental organisations (NGOs), community-based organisations (CBOs) and local health workers who seek to help break the cycle of disease transmission by improving the hygiene conditions of communities and households in developing countries. This booklet aims to assist them in developing smart hygiene promotion interventions by offering an overview of different approaches and tools that intend to improve hygiene behaviours and environmental conditions. It aims to inspire the reader to find out more about the methods and tools presented in the booklet. Like the previous booklets-- Smart Water, Sanitation, Water Harvesting, Finance and Disinfection Solutions-- it is not written to serve as a manual, but aims to provide the reader with useful links for further reading.

The first part of the booklet provides an introduction on the importance of hygiene and the concept of hygiene promotion.

The next part describes several hygiene promotion methods and highlights cases in which these methods have been used.

The final section of the booklet describes some smart tools and tips that facilitate good hygiene behaviour.

We sincerely hope that this booklet will inspire and assist people to make the right choice for smart hygiene solutions that will contribute to improve the hygiene behaviours and conditions of their target groups.

WHAT IS HYGIENE?

The importance of hygiene

The provision of safe water and sanitation is one of the keys to break the cycle of poverty. Access to safe drinking water and basic sanitation has therefore been included as a target in the Millennium Development Goals (MDGs). However, the risk is that if too much emphasis is given to the technical solutions to increase the number of people gaining access to water and sanitation, while the importance of hygiene in water and sanitation programmes is overlooked. Promoting hygiene not only contributes to improved health outcomes but is a crucial factor in the sustainability of water and sanitation programmes.

If health is the machinery of life, cleanliness is its tools and spare parts -
As'ad Khalil Dagher

Unhygienic behaviour has a tremendous impact on human health and development. Diarrhoeal diseases and pneumonia together for example, are responsible for approximately 40 per cent (3.4 million children) of all under five deaths around the world each year (UNICEF/WHO, 2009). A substantial part of this can be prevented with safe hygiene practices.

The results of an overall analysis of WASH-interventions (3IE, 2009) point out that hygienic behaviour is a vital element of the prevention of diarrhoeal diseases. It indicated that more than one out of three cases of diarrhoeal disease (37%) might be avoided in children younger than five years by consistent hand washing with soap. The same study found that improving sanitation (34%) and ensuring access to safe water at the point of use (29%) are of prime importance as well. Hygiene education on its own was related to a 27% reduction of diarrhoeal disease.

Figure 1: Effectiveness (%) of WASH interventions to reduce diarrhoea morbidity in children under 5.

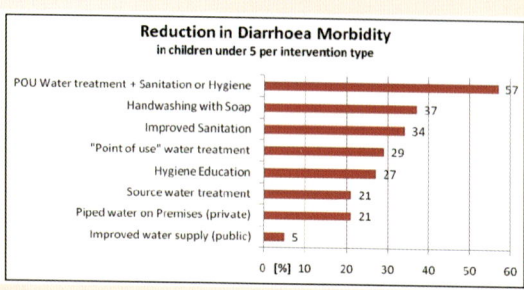

(Source: 3IE, 2009)

The positive effects of hand washing with soap are not limited to the reduction of diarrhoea. The rate of respiratory diseases was found to be almost one-fourth less (25% reduction) as a result of hand washing with soap (Ensink & Curtis). However, hygiene behaviour includes more than hand washing and its impact on people's health is therefore even greater than outlined above. Good personal and environmental hygiene for example are of prime importance for reducing blinding Trachoma, a disease currently affecting 84 million people worldwide of which 7.6 million are blind (WHO, 2005). For people suffering from HIV/AIDS, hygiene measures are very important as well. Because their resistance is lower for other diseases, people with HIV/AIDS more frequently have diarrhoea and skin infections, both of which are often waterborne and are related to poor hygiene (WSSCC, 2009).

What do we mean by hygiene?
The word *hygiene* refers to the practice of keeping oneself and one's surrounding clean, especially in order to prevent illness or the spread of disease. So, *hygiene* refers to behaviours and practices that are used to break the chain of infection transmission in the home and community. Good hygiene and sanitation practices are closely linked and often difficult to distinguish. Therefore it is important to mention that in this booklet the word *sanitation* refers to the individual management of human excreta and that sanitation in this sense is included in the concept of hygiene as defined above. The concept of hygiene can be subdivided into different categories such as personal, water, food and environmental hygiene, and is not limited to the prevention of water related diseases alone. However, because this booklet is part of a SMART Solutions Series on WASH, we will focus largely on hygienic practices that aim to prevent water borne diseases.

Transmission and prevention of water borne diseases
Water borne diseases are also called faecal-oral diseases, since they are largely caused by micro-organisms present in human or animal waste (faeces) finding their way into humans via the mouth (orally). The transmission may happen through drinking from a contaminated water supply (water-borne disease), but more often faecal –oral diseases are spread via hands, clothes, food and utensils for cooking, eating or drinking.

Water borne diseases are the main cause of diarrhoea and consequently the main focus of hygiene promotion within the field of water and sanitation.

Figure 2: The F-diagram explains the fecal-oral transmission route and barriers.

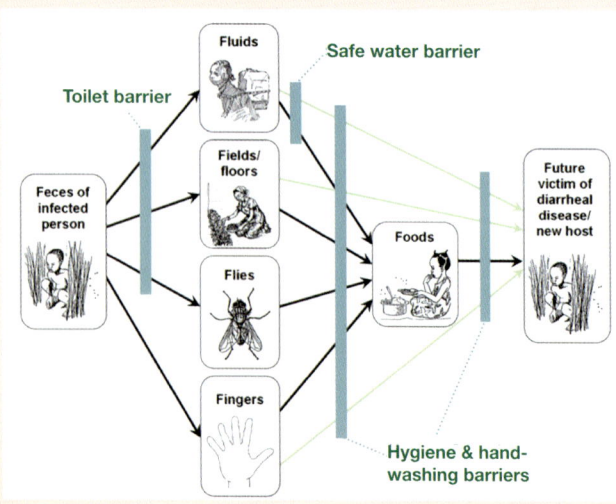

(Source: Water1st.org)

Three crucial behaviours
It is widely recognised that for reducing the risk of diarrhoeal disease transmission, great attention needs to be given to three interventions that form a barrier in the fecal-oral transmission route as shown in figure 2. These interventions are:
- Hand washing with soap at critical times
- Ensuring access to safe drinking water at the point of use
- Safe disposal of faeces

Other hygiene practices are generally introduced once these primary interventions are in place.

For the successful implementation of a hygiene promotion programme, it is important to focus on only a small number of practices at one time. Therefore it is necessary to focus on those practices that form the greatest health risk for the community. This can be difficult if the community is not particularly interested in a crucial practice. Some projects begin with hygiene or sanitation activities in which the communities and community leaders have greatest interest.

This might, for example, be cleaning public areas or building toilets. Then, the other crucial hygiene practices are gradually introduced. Some projects spend considerable time and resources on motivating people for the crucial hygiene practices in which, at first, they had less interest, for example, hand washing by men.

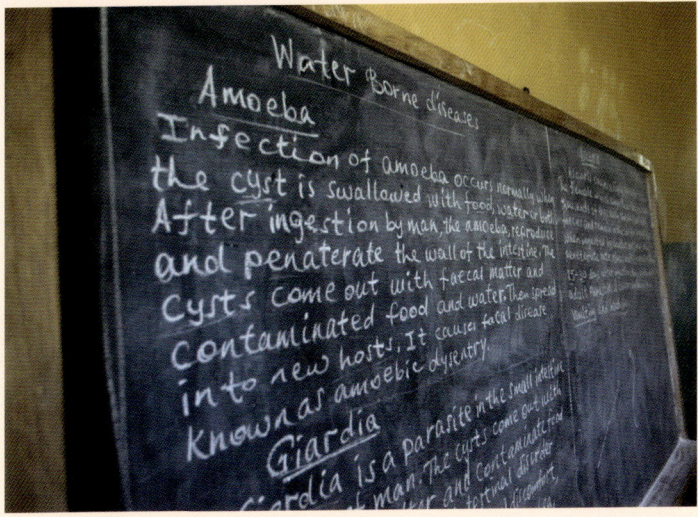

(Source: PLAN)

WHAT IS HYGIENE PROMOTION?

What do we mean by hygiene promotion
Hygiene promotion encourages people to replace their unsafe hygiene practices with simple, safe alternatives. In many parts of the developing world these practices are not traditionally seen as ways to prevent disease and therefore must be actively promoted within water and sanitation projects.

How hygiene behaviours can best be stimulated, is subject to many studies and discussions. The first generation of hygiene improvement programmes consisted of top-down communication and educational activities that mainly addressed the link between good hygiene and better health. This method is known as hygiene education. In recent years it has become clear that providing information on health alone is not sufficient to change people's practices. Knowledge is not enough. People can be strongly motivated to change their behaviour by improvements in privacy, convenience, dignity, security, social status resulting from changes in sanitation and hygiene as well as disgust with the old practices (Jenkins and Sugden, 2006). Economic savings and incentives, like lower costs for health care, can also play an important role in behavioural change. These insights have led to new approaches that, as a group, are called *hygiene promotion*. This bottom-up approach, if carried out correctly, takes into account and challenges the different reasons that motivate or hold people back from improving their hygiene behaviours. Hygiene education may be part of this methodology; however, hygiene promotion includes additional elements. Hygiene promotion builds upon the knowledge, behaviour and beliefs that people already have. Hygiene promotion for improved sanitation practices also includes a set of interventions that aim to make an end to open defecation and create demand for sanitary facilities. The phrase *sanitation promotion* refers to that particular branch.

Communication Channels for promoting Hygiene
Communication is at the heart of all smart hygiene promotion programmes. The transfer of information (communication) has an important role in making target populations aware of right hygienic practices and the benefits of investing in them. The essence of good communication is to bring across a clear message through the right communication channel for the targeted audience. It's important to not overload the audience with too much information at one time and to focus on a few messages only. There are different communication channels to use based upon the programme objective and the audience:
- **Interpersonal communication**: This is an intensive, interactive and trust provoking medium. It reaches only a small segment of the population at once.

But it is suitable for providing detailed information and helps to instantly address important issues. It facilitates the creation of a supportive environment and allows for immediate feedback. The medium is appropriate to communicate messages to an illiterate audience and can reach areas that aren't covered by mass media.

- **Traditional media**: Storytelling, folk dances, live theatre, songs etc. are traditional forms for the transfer of information and are still effective for transmitting messages. This media enables the use of local customs and terms that make it easy for the audience to relate to. It also allows for the involvement of the community. This medium reaches only a small number of individuals at the same time.
- **Graphics**: Graphics can be used to support a message, which is also delivered through another medium. When the target audience is exposed to the graphic, it acts a reminder of the message they've received before. Graphics provides basic information on the issue or the product at stake and its benefits. Graphics can also be distributed in areas that have not been reached by mass media.
- **Print mass media**: Print media is an important means for reaching a large literate number of people in one stroke. Print media is considered to be trustworthy. It is suitable for providing detailed information, but focusing on the key message is recommended for achieving optimum results. The use of visuals makes a print message more effective. Print media is only accessible for a literate audience.
- **Audiovisual mass media (radio and television)**: Can be very powerful and have the capacity of reaching a large literate and illiterate audience at once. The images visible on television or created by radio make the message more receptive and contribute to the credibility of the message as well. Communication via radio and television is suitable for both literates and illiterates.

Case Communication Channels: Radio Soap Pilika Pilika in Tanzania
Pilika Pilika is a weekly radio soap, which engages listeners in water, sanitation and hygiene issues through the characters living in the hypothetical village of Jitazame. The characters' experiences are being used to highlight behaviours detrimental to health and offer solutions to existing problems. The radio soap is backed up by a radio talk show in which listeners call or write in with questions and experts are interviewed giving practical advice on how to address problems raised in the soap opera. For example, numerous listeners write in to request information on how to prevent collapsing of latrines or instructions on how to make a Tippy Tap. The radio programme has

> national coverage and is aired at prime time when most of the rural and peri-urban communities listen to the radio.
> The Pilika Pilika radio programme focuses on communities who have little access to education and information on issues affecting their lives like health, water and education. Monitoring and evaluation reveals that the programme provides for a crucial platform for education, helping behaviour change and empowerment in rural and peri-urban communities. Water and sanitation related health problems are addressed in an easy and accessible way and the programme appears to be popular in many communities.
> (Source: Simavi)

Participatory methods

Most of the hygiene and sanitation promotion methods described in this booklet are based on participation of groups or whole communities. To stimulate this participation, different participatory methods can be used. Participatory methods are interactive and often visual which encourage the involvement of individuals in a group learning and action planning processes. They are designed to build self-esteem and a sense of responsibility for decisions.

Examples of participatory methods are focussed group discussions (if carried out correctly), community mapping and three pile sorting. With three pile sorting participants are given a set of drawings showing different situations. For example: about household hygiene practices or latrine use. They are then asked to decide in small groups whether each picture is good, bad or in-between, putting the drawings in piles according to their choice, and explaining their choices.

To understand hygiene and sanitation issues fully, it is necessary to understand why people do what they do and what physical, social, cultural or economic constraints might influence their behaviour. There are many participatory methods that can be used to gather this kind of information such as discussing the history line in a group or health walks, school surveys and key informant discussions.

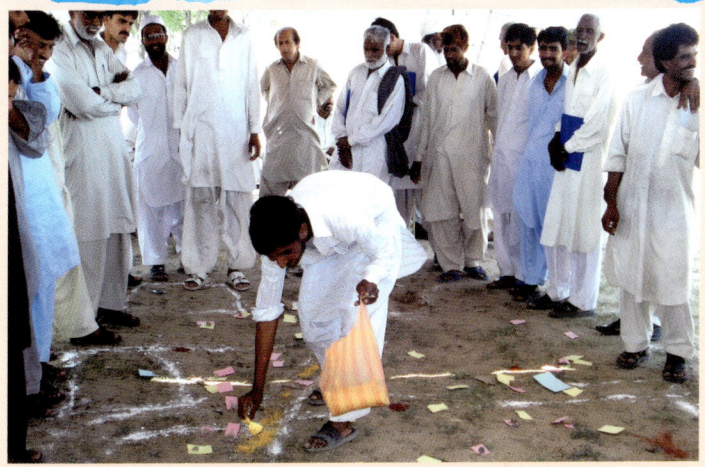
(Source: PLAN)

During a health walks a study team of people from the community walks around the town or village and marks on a map or makes a map with key information such as where people get their drinking water, the condition of pumps, and where open defecation takes place, who has toilets and so on. This information can then be used in the planning to discuss what the ideal situation would be, what needs to take place to achieve the ideal and how to change this behaviour.

The challenges of SMART hygiene promotion
Hygiene promotion is a delicate intervention because it aims to change people's behaviour that originates in local customs, taboos and beliefs. Facilitating behavioural change therefore requires an in-depth knowledge of the target community. In order to be effective, hygiene promoters need to have well-designed approaches that allow them to understand the motivations, concerns and constraints of the community with regard to hygiene behaviour. These determinants, also called enabling factors, need to be addressed in such a way that the target community itself is able to bring about and continue new healthy practices. Therefore, it is important to recognise that new behaviours are not only controlled by motivation but also by opportunities and abilities. These, in turn, are influenced by various factors such as gender, ethnicity, religion, age, setting (rural versus urban), availability of water and so on. Concerning

gender one should not only focus on women and children, but also involve men in order to have maximum impact. Because of the difference in hygiene problems and possible solutions in rural or urban settings hygiene and sanitation should be promoted differently. It is also important to consider the cost and effort required to try out a new practice. If the effort required seems too much to people (for example, a lot more water has to be taken from a distant water point), then it will be difficult to sustain a new practice.

Just as there are many challenges in hygiene promotion, so there are many approaches and methods. SMART hygiene promotion involves choosing the right methods for the community at stake and increasing their access to helpful tools and techniques. This booklet aims to assist in making a deliberate choice for SMART hygiene promotion by offering an overview of the different approaches and tools that facilitate good hygiene behaviour.

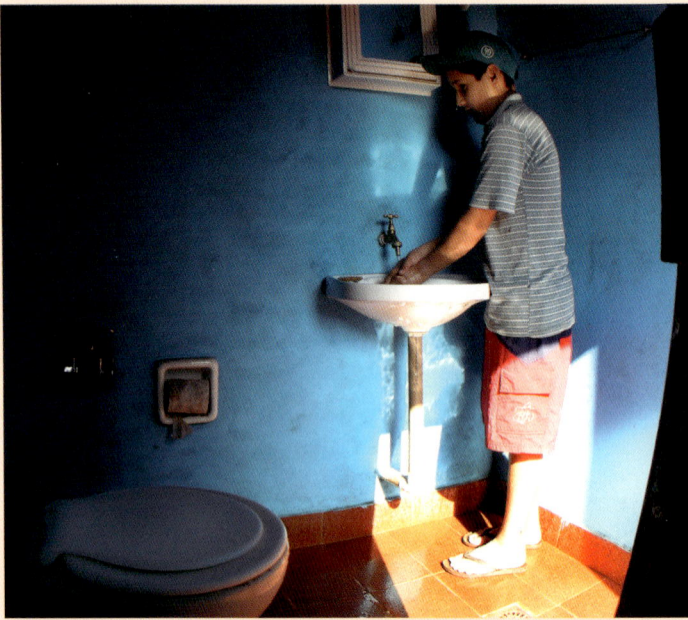

(Source: PLAN)

METHODS OF HYGIENE PROMOTION

This chapter will give some examples of methods and strategies that can be used by development workers to promote safer hygienic and sanitation practices. This chapter will provide you with a short description of the most commonly used methods, tips and pitfalls and a case where this approach has been used in practice. It is important to realize that the methods and strategies presented here are described only briefly and that the overview is not exhaustive. When handbooks and training manuals are available for a certain method or strategy, this will be mentioned in the following sections.

To promote hygiene and sanitation, there are three main approaches: participatory methods, social marketing strategies and community (and school) based strategies. These approaches overlap somewhat; and thus, a social marketing project might contain participatory activities. Similarly, a programme that is community-based can have many participatory activities or social marketing methods. What approaches or strategies are most suitable for a certain hygiene promotion programme depends on the local conditions and specific objectives of that programme and should be carefully planned by the implementing actors. It may be helpful to understand the improvement of hygiene behaviours and sanitation as a process, sometimes compared to a ladder. With respect to sanitation, people are expected to move along a continuum from open defecation via improved facilities to the use of private hygienic toilets. On the hygiene ladder people are expected to follow a continuum that ranges from no key behaviours at all to achieving a fully hygienic environment in the end. Both processes are depicted in figure 4.

Figure 3: The Hygiene and Sanitation ladder.

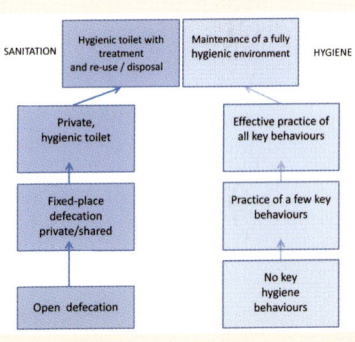

(Source: WSCC, 2010)

Most of the time, these processes do not move step-by-step. Instead of moving up the ladder one step at the time, communities and households will move up and down and skip steps as circumstances dictate. It is the task of the people involved in projects to select interventions that respond to the current set of behaviours in the community and seek to make sustainable moves up the ladder. This booklet aims to provide information to help make these decisions.

PARTICIPATORY STRATEGIES

Participatory Hygiene and Sanitation Transformation (PHAST)

What is it?
Participatory Hygiene and Sanitation Transformation (PHAST) is designed to promote hygiene behaviour, sanitation improvement and community management of water and sanitation facilities. It does so by promoting health awareness and understanding which leads to environmental and behavioural improvements. PHAST builds on people's ability to address and resolve their own problems via participatory learning.

How does it work?
PHAST uses methods and materials that stimulate the participation of women, men and children in the development process. The materials comprise of a series of images that refer to hygiene circumstances. Groups of people from the community are asked to relate these images to the local situation and to share how they feel this situation should be addressed. People are not provoked to expose themselves and share their private experiences. When individual input is required a method is available that allows the participants to vote in secret (see page 28 for more information on Community Health Clubs).

PHAST uses seven steps to facilitate community planning and action:
1. Problem identification
2. Problem analyses
3. Planning for solutions
4. Selecting options
5. Planning for new facilities and behaviour change
6. Planning for monitoring end evaluation
7. Participatory evaluation

When to Use it?
The PHAST method can be used in communities where basic hygiene behaviour and/or sanitation facilities are lacking or not entirely developed. PHAST can be used in both rural and urban areas. The method can be adjusted to deal with HIV/AIDS, alcohol and drug abuse as well. PHAST has been successfully used within Community Health Clubs.

Tips & Pitfalls
- PHAST is about facilitation and not about directing. Communities should determine their own priorities for disease prevention.
- Skilled and trained facilitators are needed for PHAST. Community members must invest time in the PHAST exercises.
- PHAST method has a tendency to become a talk shop. Make sure that plans reach the implementation phase.
- PHAST relies heavily on graphic materials (toolkits) that should be produced locally to suit the local circumstances.
- When financial resources are limited one can make good use of cheaper toolkits, for example by bringing along paper and colouring pencils and let the community make their own drawings.

Case PHAST: Katwe Urban Pilot Project, Uganda
In Uganda PHAST has been tested in the Katwe Urban Pilot Project (KUPP) in a low-income peri-urban artisan community near the city of Kampala. Here, five extension workers and 20 community members were trained in the methods.
The project goal was to improve environmental conditions by using the PHAST method to stimulate community involvement, to raise awareness about health risks and to set in motion some planning and action. At first the community, mostly men, was resistant even to meet with field workers. However, little by little, community members began attending meetings and using the graphic materials to discuss their problems.
Within six months of an initial visit by one field worker, the community built latrines, organized the operation and maintenance of neglected communal drains, collected tariffs to pay for maintenance workers for drains and water points, and organized their own system of monitoring community sanitation. The community adopted the graphic materials and discussion techniques of the field worker in order to continue the process of community development in her absence.
(Source: WHO)

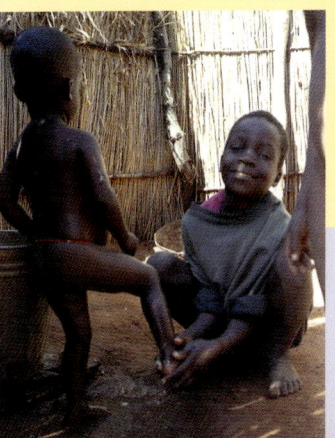

Further Reading
Download PHAST manual on:
http://www.who.int/water_sanitation_health/hygiene/envsan/phastep/en/index.html

PARTICIPATORY STRATEGIES

Children's Hygiene And Sanitation Training (CHAST) & Participatory Hygiene and Sanitation Education (PHASE)

What is it?
Because the PHAST approach was initially designed for adults, it has been revised and adapted to suit the needs of young children. Both the Children's Hygiene And Sanitation Training (CHAST) and the Participatory Hygiene and Sanitation Education (PHASE) approach are based on the premise that personal hygiene practices are usually acquired during childhood, and that it is much easier to change the habits of children than those of adults. While children have less knowledge and experience, fewer responsibilities and a different perception of time and the future, they are also naturally inquisitive and eager to learn. The CHAST and PHASE materials take advantage of these natural attributes. CHAST and PHASE encourage children to actively participate in open discussions and, wherever possible, to share their experiences and ideas with other children and their family. CHAST does this in a community environment and PHASE in a school environment.

How does it work?
In the CHAST/PHASE exercises, children are encouraged to work independently in pairs or in small groups, and then to present their thoughts and findings to the larger group. Above all, CHAST/PHASE tools are meant to be fun, involving games, exercises and role-plays that prompt the children to discuss and genuinely understand the key issues related to personal cleanliness and hygiene.

Step-by-step activities:
1. Introduction/warming up
2. Problem identification
3. Problem analyses
4. Practicing good behaviour
5. Monitoring/ reflection/ follow up

When to use it?
PHASE can be used within schools where basic hygiene behaviour and/or sanitation facilities are lacking or not entirely developed. CHAST/PHASE can be used in both rural and urban-based settings. School Health (Hygiene) Clubs should be introduced as part of the approach (see page 30 for more information on School Health Clubs).

Tips & Pitfalls
- If schools don't provide the facilities children need for sanitation, hand washing and water supply it may be very difficult for the children to acquire appropriate sanitation and hygiene behaviour.
- Emphasis is not on instruction but on challenging the children to think for themselves and to facilitate them towards decision making.
- Continuing maintenance and provision for purchase of materials (soap, cleansing materials, spare parts) should be planned carefully from the beginning.

Case PHASE: David Wamalwa, former PHASE Project Manager AMREF:
When we started the project in 1998 in the four pilot schools in Western Kenya, we discovered that the performance of students improved considerably and cases of absenteeism had reduced significantly. All this because of the simple awareness of the importance of cleaning your hands! We called it 'happy hands'.
Armed with the results from the pilot schools, in 2000 PHASE was scaled up to 247 schools in 10 districts in Kenya, reaching approximately 83,000 children. PHASE also helped increase the use of tippy taps, latrines, dish racks and refuse pits, and the treatment of water in the target communities. This helped us identify the three pillars of PHASE: hand washing, greater access to water and safer human waste disposal. Apart from school health clubs, information was also transmitted through the Child to Parent component of PHASE. Pupils trained at school went back home and passed information on hygiene and sanitation to their parents and their community. The project also included de-worming and construction of toilets and hand washing points at schools.

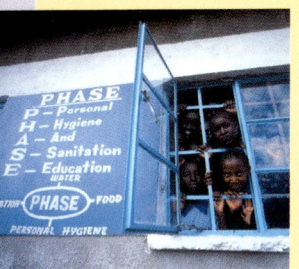

By the end of the project in 2004, absenteeism, diarrhoea, cases of intestinal worms and eye and skin infections had greatly reduced in schools practising PHASE, compared with those that did not.
In 2009 the Ministry of Education also developed and launched, what it calls the 'Comprehensive School Health Policy' that is based on PHASE experiences and lessons learned. (Source: AMREF)

Further Reading
- Download CHAST manual on:
  http://ochaonline.un.org/OchaLinkClick.aspx?link=ocha&docId=1108772
- Download Children's Hygiene And Sanitation Training (CHAST): A practical guide: www.schools.watsan.net/Somalia%20ofinal%20%20CHAST%20SSHE%20case%20 study_WE...
- Website about WASH in Schools: http://www.schools.watsan.net
- Website Children's Hygiene And Sanitation Training (CHAST) in Somalia: http://www.irc.nl/page/13170

SOCIAL MARKETING

What is it?
Social marketing, developed in retail businesses, became a strategy for hygiene programming about 20 years ago. Marketing requires an understanding of what the target audience wants. People have many competing priorities in life and the behaviour being promoted needs to be perceived as a top priority. The target audience must want and be able to change their behaviour. Social marketing is developed around a "4P" framework:

1. Product may be an object (like a latrine) or a practice with objects (e.g. washing hands with soap).
2. Price: Products need to be affordable in terms of money and the extra effort needed, for example, effort to carry more water home.
3. Place: The products must be easily available and communication must reach the audiences.
4. Promotion requires understanding the motivations of audiences and the channels of communication they trust.

How does it work?
There are five major stages in social marketing:

1. Planning: Define the desired behaviour. Break the target audience into groups that will be reached in different ways such as mothers of young children or fathers. Study the barriers and motivations for changing behaviour and how to communicate this.
2. Plan different messages for each audience, for example, disgust with contamination or desire to care for children or dignity. Study how to reach the different audiences (radio, face-to-face communication, schools, etc.).
3. Pre-test and select the messages and ways of reaching the audiences.
4. Implementation: Bring together partners, train, produce materials/programmes, implement as planned.
5. Monitoring: Measure access to messages, frequency, problems and behaviour change taking place. Change the plan when monitoring shows there are problems.

When to use it?
Single and not too complex hygiene practices, such as hand washing with soap at critical times or hygienic use of toilets may be promoted best through social marketing approaches.

Tips & Pitfalls
Use formative research to develop the programme, including in-depth interviews, focus group discussions and surveys, and trials with small groups.
- Social marketing of hand washing with soap has grown internationally mainly in large-scale programmes. NGOs can apply the same approaches at local levels, using a combination of local media and inter-personal contacts.

Case Social Marketing: Promoting hand washing with soap in Vietnam
The Water and Sanitation Program (WSP) has supported the Ministries of Health and Education to carry out a social marketing programme promoting hand washing with soap among women aged 15-49 and schoolchildren aged 6-10 in Vietnam. Research was conducted with mothers and school children, teachers and also grandparents who also take care of grandchildren. This gave insight into the minds and realities of caregivers and children to better understand barriers and motivations to washing hands with soap. For children, the research led to an education entertainment programme combining mass media and interpersonal communications to reach children in the classrooms and in their homes. For women, promotion of hand washing with soap is done through journals, television, and interpersonally by the national women's and youth unions. These organisations have influence and are respected. The programme has reached almost two million people up to 2010 and will expand.
(Source WSP)

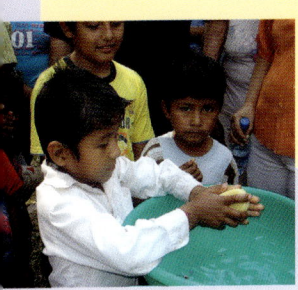

(Source: PLAN)

Further Reading
- Download WELL factsheets: the process of sanitation marketing: http://www.lboro.ac.uk/well/resources/fact-sheets/fact-sheets-htm/Sanitation%20marketing.htm
- Download WELL Factsheet Social Marketing: A Consumer-based Approach to Promoting Safe Hygiene Behaviours: http://www.ilboro.ac.uk/well/resources/fact-sheets/fact-sheets-htm/Social%20marketing.htm
- Website Unilevers hand washing campaign: www.lifebuoy.com
- Website Global Handwashing Partnership: http://globalhandwashing.org/

Community Led Total Sanitation (CLTS)

What is it?
Community Led Total Sanitation (CLTS) is a sanitation promotion strategy that focuses on igniting a change in sanitation behaviour. CLTS focuses on the dangers of open defecation and emphasizes the sense of disgust about this practice. Social solidarity, help and cooperation among the households in the community are a common and vital element in CLTS.

How does it work?
The goal of CLTS is for communities to reach the Open Defecation Free (ODF) status. While there is considerable variation among CLTS programmes, the approach usually includes the following steps:
1. Discuss the impacts of open defecation with an external facilitator.
2. Visit sites of open defecation by community members and leaders.
3. Map out the areas of open defecation.
4. Work out how much human waste they produce in total.
5. The community draws up an action plan to tackle the situation.
6. Health and hygiene promotion sessions are carried out.
7. The facilitator and community work out an action plan.
8. Construction of latrines begins[1]. Members of the community who are not abiding by the new rules are discouraged from this behaviour.
9. Latrines are now available to everyone and hygiene promotion continues.
10. The community is awarded ODF status and a sign is erected at the entrance of the village.

When to Use it?
CLTS is used in areas where open defecation is a common practice. CLTS is easier to launch in communities that have not been previously reached by other hygiene or sanitation interventions. When subsidies have been involved earlier, people may have reservations about the CLTS approach. CLTS has been developed for rural areas. However, efforts are being made to adjust CLTS to urban settings[2].

---

[1] In the ignition phase, emphasis is on reaching ODF status and thus on the quantity of latrines. In a later stage the quality of latrines needs to be addressed, for example by means of a social marketing campaign.

[2] PLAN International has conducted a pilot on Urban Total Sanitation (UTS) in Bangladesh and is currently starting up UTS in African Countries.

Tips & Pitfalls
- It is fundamental that CLTS involves no individual hardware subsidies and does not prescribe latrine models.
- Learn local, crude words for 'shit' and use them to cut through the deadly silence around open defecation.
- Emphasis on social control should not lead to harsh punishment of people who do not participate.
- It is important to emphasise on practices such as cleaning and sustaining latrines.

Case Community Led Total Sanitation: How to say shit in Portuguese

"How do you say 'shit'?" asks UNICEF WASH specialist Americo Muianga. Huge giggles erupt from the crowd, along with the answer, "matudzi."

Volunteers are drawn from the crowd to draw a map of their village. In Chibwe, the villagers use a stick to outline the roads and houses in the sand. White maize powder defines the major landmarks: the school, the water point, the road to the nearest clinic, the local church. More volunteers are asked to stand where they live. From there they are given grey ash and asked to mark where they defecate. Embarrassed chuckles follow as piles of grey ash appear on the map.

"You then calculate the quantity of faeces for each week, month and year for each household," says Mr. Muianga. "Then you start discussing the quantity and where it goes." The tabulation is drawn on white butcher paper and held up for everyone to see – 84,720 piles of faeces annually from 93 households. The giggles become laughs. Then begins the 'walk of shame' in which village members are asked to physically go to where the excreta is and see how it could infect the local water supply or contribute to breeding grounds for flies and mosquitoes. They return to the shade of the trees for a food demonstration. A plate of fresh food is given to a volunteer to eat. After a few mouthfuls, the plate is put in the centre of the crowd, along with some just-collected faeces. It does not take long in the heat for the flies to move back and forth between the two. Asked to resume eating, the volunteer quickly refuses, shaking his head in horror. No one chuckles. They get it.
(Source: Unicef)

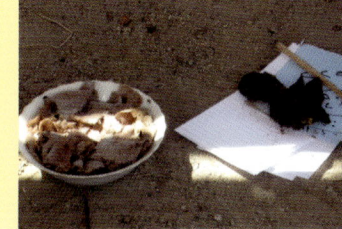
(Source: PLAN)

Further Reading
- Download Handbook on CLTS (IDS and Plan International): http://www.communityledtotalsanitation.org/resource/handbook-community-led-total-sanitation
- Website CLTS: http://www.communityledtotalsanitation.org

School Led Total Sanitation

What is it?
School Led Total Sanitation (SLTS) is a variation or an addition to the Community Led Total Sanitation (CLTS) method. In the SLTS method schools serve as centers for change in the communities. School children bring home the lessons learned on toilet use and hygiene behaviour and influence their families and other children in the community.

The distinction between SLTS and Child Hygiene and Sanitation Training (CHAST) is that SLTS focuses on the community via school children and emphasizes the dangers of open defecation and a sense of disgust. CHAST focuses on children and not on the community. Above all CHAST tools are meant to be fun.

How does it work?
The approach is built on the use of activity-oriented, participatory exercises to raise awareness of sanitation issues among school children. Hygiene education and CLTS-type sanitation promotion tools are used to encourage children to change their hygiene and sanitation behaviour. As the process unfolds the school environment becomes cleaner; the adults then see the improvements at the school and instigate changes at home. Therefore, the children become agents of change as their school leads the way in promotion of sanitation improvements within their community (WSSCC, 2010).

When to use it
SLTS can be used in situations where open defecation is still common and/or toilets are not yet available in a community.

> **Tips & Pitfalls**
> - The success of the approach depends heavily upon the teachers training and motivation. The teachers must be motivated to take a leading role.
> - Preferably teachers should live in the community rather than on the school campus. In this way the teachers will also bring the sanitation issue into the community.
> - SLTS is can also be combined with Community Led Total Sanitation.
> - (see CLTS for more tips & pitfalls).

Case SLTS: School Children lead sanitation drive in Nepal

Around the countryside of the Kaski district in Nepal, school children led their communities in a sanitation drive as the Eighth National Sanitation Action Week got underway earlier this month. All 549 homes in the area of this Village Development Committee have a toilet and there is no open defecation.

"Earlier when we went to our neighbours and told them about the benefits of constructing a latrine, they would chase us out as if we said something offensive," says eighth grader Madan Pokharel, the chairperson of the children's club for Meghraj Lower Secondary School. "But now, everybody takes pride in the fact that there isn't even cow-dung or trash on the roads in our village," says the 14-year-old. "The children were excited when we told them what we were planning to do in the village," says Tika Ram Lamsal, the headmaster of Meghraj Lower Secondary School and coordinator of the total sanitation campaign for Ghachowk village. "We did all we could but it was ultimately upon children like Madan who could better convince their parents," he says. Initially, UNICEF and the Water Supply and Sanitation Sub Divisional Office (WSSDO) trained the teachers and offered to provide a toilet pan, pipes and technical support to every household to construct a latrine. But soon, community members started buying their own materials, and now most donor agencies are discouraging any direct interventions.

After the school students received training from their teachers, they began to campaign and educate their parents and neighbours about the benefits of constructing a latrine and keeping their community clean. The joint committee of students and adult community members also share responsibilities for trash collection, sweeping roads and clearing the neighbourhood of animal waste.
(Source: Unicef)

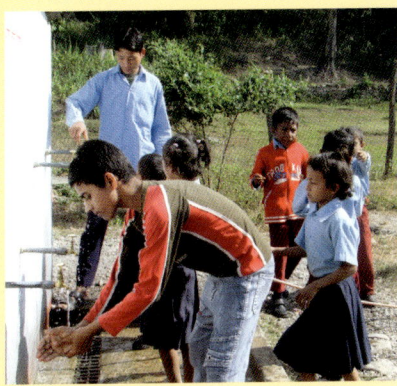

(Source: Unicef)

Further Reading
- Download Guidelines on School Led Total Sanitation. Steering Committee for National Sanitation Action Department of Water Supply and Sewerage and UNICEF, Nepal (2006): http://origin-www.unicef.org/wash/files/SLTS_Book_(Eng).pdf
- SLTS information on website IRC: http://www.irc.nl/page/40584

Community Health (Hygiene) Clubs

What is it?
Community Health Clubs (CHC) are free, voluntary, community-based organisations formed to provide a forum for information and good practice relating to improving family health. They vary in size and composition and are facilitated by a health extension worker. The concept of a CHC combines participatory health education with the strength of peer pressure and the desire to conform. While CHCs are meant to address health issues in general, sanitation and hygiene behaviour can be starting points for all CHCs.

How does it work?
The CHC gathers regularly and discusses health improvement opportunities that can be applied at home directly. This can involve changes like covering stored water or building a latrine with locally available materials. In the following meeting the activities and results will be discussed and if no problems arise from this appraisal a new issue will be discussed.

When to use it?
Community Health Clubs can be introduced in order to facilitate the implementation of PHAST, CLTS and other forms of hygiene and health promotion activities.

> **Tips & Pitfalls**
> - More than one CHC can be organized in a community.
> - Mobilisation by political, religious and local leaders is a key factor for the successful creation of CHCs.
> - Membership cards and attendance certificates are important incentives for members.
> - Opportunities for income generation may be another incentive for members to join the CHC.
> - Community peer pressure and the member's desire to conform to social norms are paramount for the success of the CHC.
> - Organise meetings at most convenient time and location for all members.

Case Community Health Club: Uganda
In Pader district, a hygiene and sanitation promotion project has been implemented by an NGO called Health Integrated Development Organisation based in Gulu district. The aim of the project was promoting sanitation and hygiene in nine satellite camps where internally displaced people live.

Some of the CHC activities include: home improvement activities like digging latrines, refuse pits, bath shelters and drying racks, formation of drama groups within the clubs, inter- and intra-club competitions. Some of the achievements over a period of two months in the nine camps were the construction of sanitation facilities in large numbers: 500 pit latrines, 108 rubbish pits, 1223 drying racks, 228 hand washing facilities and 658 bath shelters.
(Source: IRC)

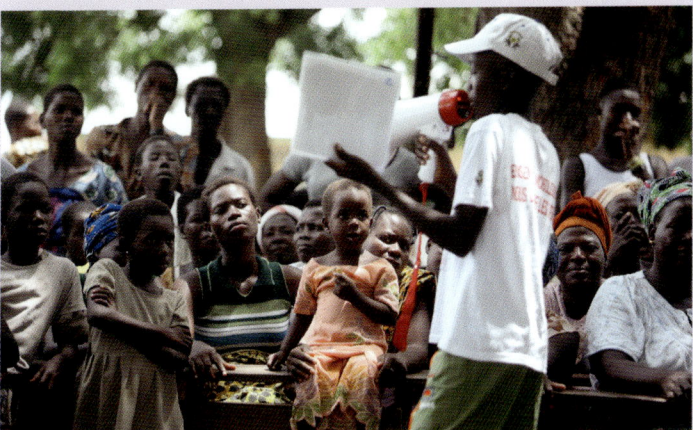

(Source: PLAN)

Further Reading
- Download factsheets that can be used as education material within clubs: http://www.connectinternational.nl/english/smartmodules/smart-dev/fact-sheets, or http://www.cawst.org/en/resources/pubs/category/1-cawst-poster-series
- WELL Briefing Note 38 (2007). The Consensus Approach. Health Promotion Through Community Health Clubs http://www.lboro.ac.uk/well/resources/Publications/Briefing%20Notes/BN%2038%20Consensus.htm
- Website Community Health Club Approach: http://www.africaahead.org/

CLUBS

School Health Clubs (SHCs)

What is it?
School Health Clubs (SHCs) support the implementation of WASH programmes in schools. The aim of SHCs is to involve children as advocates for hygiene and sanitation practices in schools and the community. The formation of a SHC offers the possibility of more interaction and participation than traditional top-down teaching. It is therefore considered to be more effective for fostering behavioural change. The concept of SHCs stems from the increasing recognition of children as effective agents of change in the area of health and hygiene.

How does it work?
SHCs exist in many forms. For example: they may be part of a children's parliament or school councils, they can be organized during school time and be led by a teacher, or be organized as a peer-to-peer activity. The members of a SHC may not only act as advocates for hygiene behaviour, but can also help to ensure that water and sanitation facilities in the schools are used and maintained properly. The members of the SHC may be in charge of water collection, organise hand washing before eating and organise the cleaning of facilities. Members of the SHC can also take part in public awareness campaigns,

When to use it?
SHCs can be usefully linked to other strategies. They can be established in order to facilitate CHAST/PHASE, CLTS and other types of hygiene and health promotion activities in schools.

> **Tips & Pitfalls**
> - SHCs with volunteers are often more motivated than clubs with appointed members.
> - A SHC should consist of a representative group from the school population.
> - Be careful to not confirm traditional gender roles by only having girls take care of the toilets.
> - Be careful to not put a too heavy burden on the members of the SHCs and be aware of the risk that members of the health club may be exploited as cheap cleaning labour.
> - The support of teachers is crucial for the existence of SHCs. Invest in teacher's motivation, knowledge and capacities. Motivate the school inspectorate and educational managers.
> - It is recommended to first concentrate on the improvement or construction of the facilities. If facilities can hardly be used or maintained, a SHC will lose its motivation.
> - Have follow-up visits from the NGO to the schools after the end of the project period to help ensure sustainability.

Case School Health Clubs: Indonesia

Plan Indonesia has a WASH project that includes schools and school hygiene. One of the objectives focuses on hygiene education outreach to children, as agents for behavioural change. In the project areas, school children try to motivate other children, individuals and families to adopt hygiene practices. The project organized School Health Clubs, in which students play the role of health worker and check on the other students. The role of the health worker rotates between the different students. The students check each other for instance on clean teeth and observe hand washing practices. When at home, children act as agents of change and catalyse their families and friends. Another part of the project is the publication of "Percik Junior". This is a free magazine for children. It was a group of children who thought of the idea, and children write many of the articles. But there's one big difference from other youth magazines: the articles are all about water, sanitation and personal hygiene. The magazine is regularly distributed in children clubs and schools in the communities. The magazines include information and experiences from children about clean water, healthy environment and good health habits. Earlier publications have focused, for instance, on saving water, garbage treatment, hand washing with soap and personal hygiene. More children are motivated to practice good health habits in school and at home and other members of their families are starting to learn good health habits.
(Source: PLAN Indonesia)

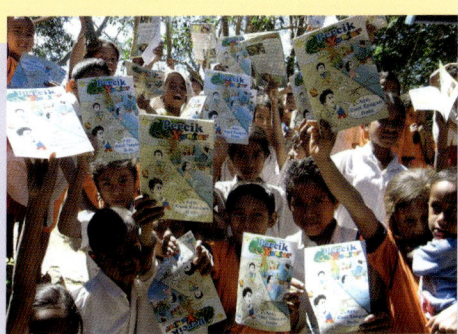

(Source: PLAN)

Further Reading
- Download songs about hygiene: http://www.irc.nl/page/26444
- Website about WASH in Schools: http://www.schools.watsan.net
- Websites Unicef about WASH in Schools:
  http://www.unicef.org/wash/schools/index.html &
  http://www.unicef.org/wash/schools/files/raisingcleanhands_2010.pdf

TOOLS ANDS TIPS FOR HYGIENE IMPROVEMENT

Sustainable changes in hygiene behaviour are not only fostered by changes in knowledge and feelings about the importance of hygiene, but also depend on the knowledge and the availability of appropriate tools and practices that facilitate this behaviour.

As mentioned earlier in this booklet, the three crucial hygiene behaviours are: hand washing with soap, ensuring access to safe drinking water at the point of use and safe disposal of faeces. In the following chapter several tools and tips for these three interventions will be described.

Because this booklet is part of a SMART solutions series on WASH, some additional hygiene tools and tips that relate to the provision of clean water and environmental sanitation are explained as well, including the management of waste water and food hygiene.

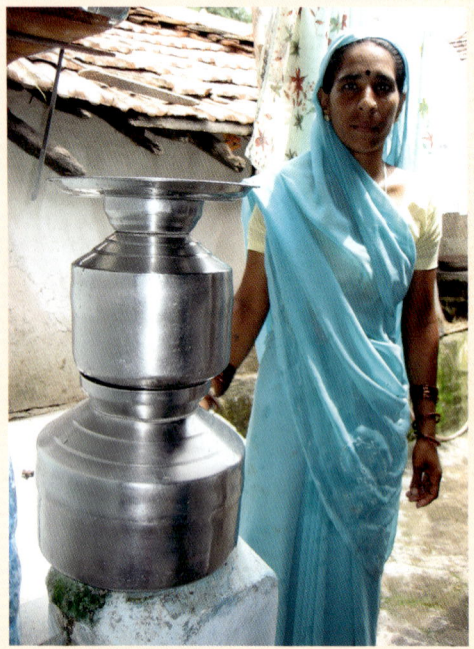

(Source: IRC)

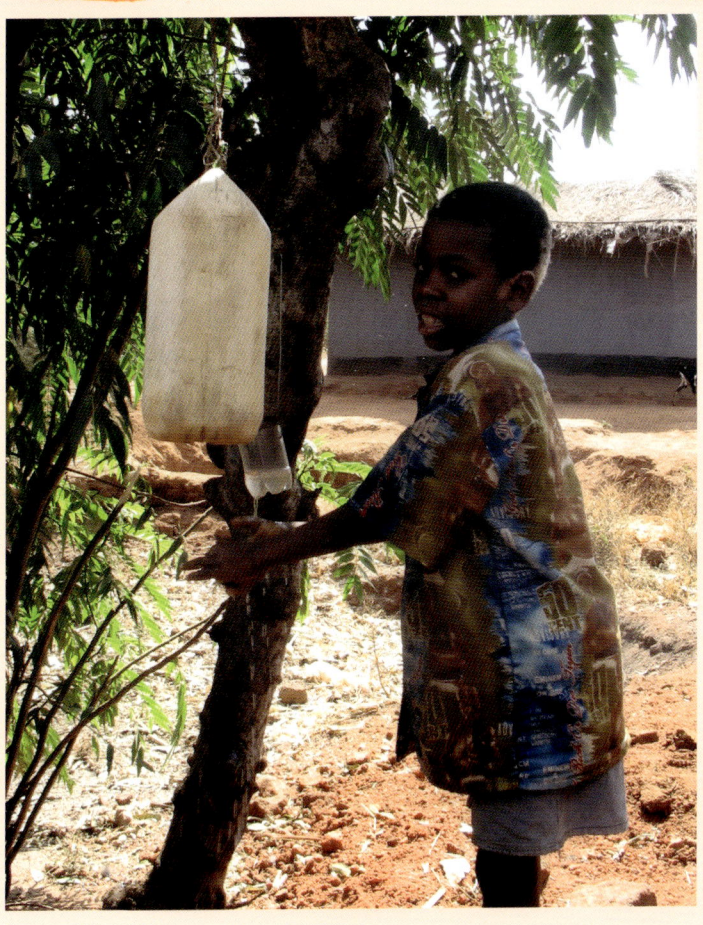
(Source: IRC)

HAND WASHING

Why is it necessary?
Hand washing with soap is one of the most important ways to prevent the spread of infection and is the single most effective way of reducing diarrhoeal illnesses: washing hands the correct way at the right times can reduce diarrhoea by nearly 40%. Hand washing can also help to reduce respiratory problems by 25%, according to a study conducted jointly by UNICEF and the World Health Organization.

What is good behaviour?
When to wash hands
It is commonly accepted that there are critical points at which you must wash your hands – these are universal, not merely depending on the location:
- After defecating and preferably also after urinating / using the toilet.
- After cleaning children's bottoms.
- Before preparing food.
- Before eating food.

The aim is to ensure hand washing with soap at each, not some, of these critical points.

How to wash hands correctly:
- Pour a bit of water on both hands.
- Put soap on hands.
- Rub hands well, at least three times all over (see below).
- Rinse well – rinsing away all of the soap.

Figure 4: How to wash hands correctly (2).

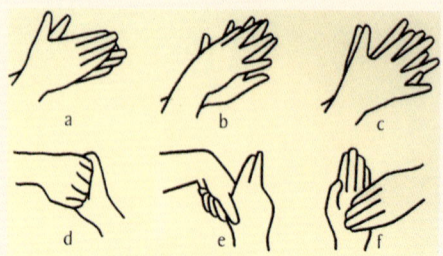

Globally around 1,500,000 to 1,700,000 lives could be saved every year by promoting hand washing with soap after contact with human excreta.

It is sometimes said that some people do not have access to soap. This is true, although it is not as frequent a problem as might be thought. Most households have soap, even if it is often for washing clothes only. Where soap simply isn't available, using a substance like ash is a reasonable substitute; however, the goal is universal use of soap.

Example Smart Hand washing Devices: The Tippy Tap
Lack of access to both piped water supply and soap, especially in schools, is a barrier to hand washing in the developing world. Various smart hand washing devices, made with commonly available materials, have been developed to overcome this problem. The Tippy Tap is one of these devices.

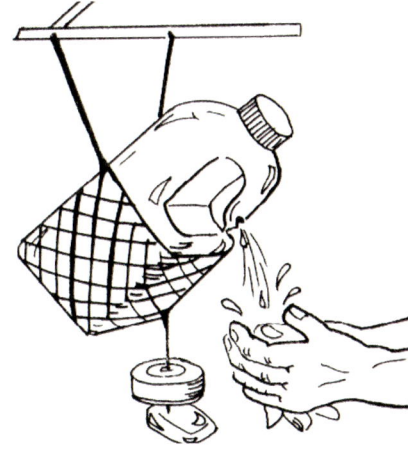

Figure 5: Tippy tap.

(Source: IRC)

Further Reading
- Download WSP Enabling Technologies for Hand Washing with Soap Database: http://www.wsp.org/wsp/global-initiatives/Global-Scaling-Up-Handwashing-Project/Enabling%20Technologies%20for%20Handwashing%20with%20Soap
- Download: 'Beyond tippy-taps: the role of enabling products in scaling up and sustaining handwashing'. Written by Jacqueline Devine for the South Asia Hygiene practitioners' workshop, 1 – 4 February 2010, Dhaka, Bangladesh. http://www.irc.nl/page/51606
- Website with information on the Tippy-Tap: http://www.akvo.org/wiki/index.php/Tippy_Tap
- Website on how to build a Tippy-Tap: http://www.wot.utwente.nl/publications/tippy-tap.pdf
- Website UNICEF Water, Environment and Sanitation Technical Guidelines Series: Hygiene Promotion Manual. New York http://www.unicef.org/wes/files/hman.pdf

SAFE EXCRETA DISPOSAL

Why is it necessary?
One gram of excreta can contain: 10,000,000 viruses, 1,000,000 bacteria, 1,000 parasite cysts and 100 parasite eggs. Even a small dose of excreta, transmitted via fingers, flies, food or water, can make a person sick. If people defecate in the open, or too close to a water source, their entire community is exposed to the danger of infection and illness.

Many people believe that excrement of children is less dangerous than that of adults. But all faeces contain small germs that can cause diseases in both children and adults. Safe excreta disposal for adults and children is therefore of prime importance for improving public health.

What is good behaviour?
Human excreta should be completely removed from human contact throughout the sanitation system (collection, transport and treatment). The use of a latrine is the most important method to separate human excreta safely from human contact in the first phase of the sanitation system. However other methods are also possible. See the Smart Sanitation Solutions booklet for other possibilities.

It is important to construct a latrine that is easy to use, clean and maintain. This means that:
- The surface of latrine slabs needs to be smooth and easy to clean
- The distance between the footsteps and the drop hole needs to be appropriate in order to prevent the slab from becoming filthy.
- There should be ventilation, with openings in the walls or a space between the roof and the walls.
- If applicable: the walls of the latrine should be plastered at least some distance from the floor to make cleaning easier.
- Prevent flies from entering by having a tight-fitting lid to close the drop hole after use, a water-trap (P-trap). Catch flies through a screened, black painted ventilation pipe exposed to the sunIf needed, add sawdust or ashes after use to prevent the breeding of flies.
- Clean regularly with a broom and/or with water and detergent.
- It is recommended to always wear footgear when using a latrine.

Example Excreta Disposal: The Peepoo Bag

The absence of hygienic sanitation facilities poses an enormous problem for the residents of poor urban areas. Usually the living areas of the poor are not covered by any urban sewerage plan and are overcrowded, which makes it impossible to construct separate household latrines. The presence of public facilities may offer some relief, but these facilities are often over-crowded, filthy or are so badly maintained that they don't offer a hygienic solution. The absence of sanitary facilities forces people to defecate in the open, or to use a 'flying toilet' (a plastic bag that is thrown outside).

The Peepoo bag is a biodegradable plastic bag with a thin inner tube that is designed to be used once for defecation and urination. Because of its design a used Peepoo is clean to handle. Next to that a Peepoo is odour free for about 12-24 hours after use. Each bag contains urea, which destroys the pathogens within 2-4 weeks and makes the excreta safe to use as a fertilizer within a relatively short period of time. The value of the fertilizer will be used to bear the costs of the collection and distribution service. The introduction of the Peepoo bag has met with a wide range of reactions, from offensive to hesitant to enthusiastic. The most frequent criticism is that the Peepoo bag is still just a plastic bag, which does not contribute to human dignity. In response the people behind Peepoo emphasise that the Peepoo is not meant to be a permanent solution, but provides a contemporary solution for as long as people are deprived of any alternative method for hygienic sanitation.

The Peepoo bag finds itself in its inception phase and is still working on improvements of the concept. The product has been launched on a small scale in Kenya and Bangladesh. The first results are encouraging.
(Source, Peepoo)

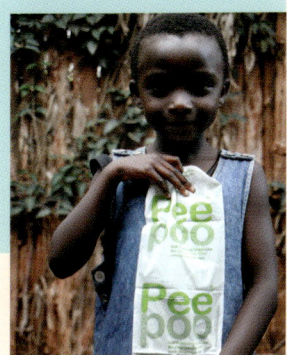

(Source: Peepoo)

Further Reading
- Download Compendium of Sanitation Systems and Technologies (EAWAG): http://www.eawag.ch/organisation/abteilungen/sandec/publikationen/publications_sesp/downloads_sesp/compendium_high.pdf
- Website with information about the Peepoo bag: www.peepoople.com
- Website with information about different sanitation options: Smart Sanitation Solutions (2006) http://www.irc.nl/page/28448

CLEAN WATER: TREATMENT, SAFE STORAGE AND ATTRACTION

Why is it necessary?
A lot of people in developing countries do not have access to safe drinking water supplies. They rely on open surface water or on wells that are not properly constructed. As a result they run the risk of using water that is contaminated. Even in case of a piped water supply, the water may not be safe. Treatment of water at household level is therefore an important measure to improve the access to safe water. But improving the quality of water alone is not sufficient. Drinking water can become contaminated after collection, either during transport or storage at the home. This recontamination often comes from inadequate storage vessels, water ladles that are contaminated by the surface where ladles rest, and direct contact with hands or animals.

What is good behaviour?
The recommended strategy for improving household drinking water combines two elements: water disinfection at the time of water collection or time of use and prevention of recontamination by safe storage.

Water disinfection
There are many methods and products available for the disinfection of contaminated water. Currently, chlorination at the source and boiling water at home are the most common methods of disinfection. But many alternatives for water treatment are available. The booklet Smart Disinfections Solutions from this Smart Solutions Series gives a broad overview of available alternatives for water disinfection.

Safe storage
Safe storage requires that water containers are designed according to the following criteria:
- Are made of a material that is durable, non-oxidizing, lightweight, easy to clean, inexpensive and preferably locally produced.
- Hold appropriate standard volumes and preferably have volume indicators for right use of disinfectants.
- Have a narrow opening that makes it easy to fill the container and add disinfectant, but prohibits dipping of hands or other utensils.
- Have a strong, tight-fitting lid.
- Water is poured out of the container, not dipped.
- Taps (if present) should be of non-rusting and durable material and be easy to clean.
- Are non translucent or stored in a dark place to prevent the growth of algae and bacteria.

- Are culturally acceptable.
- Have to be clean and disinfected before use.

Figure 6: The wrong and the right way to store water.

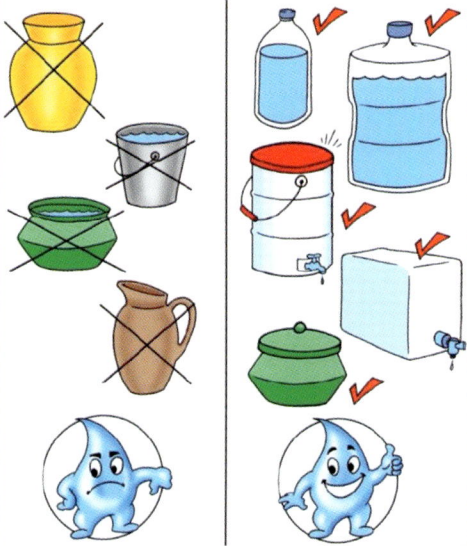

(Source: CAWST)

Further Reading
- Download Smart Disinfection Solutions (2010): http://www.kitpublishers.nl/smart-site.shtml?id=33740&ItemID=2842&ch=FAB
- Download Mintz, E., Reiff, F. & Tauxe, R. (1995). Safe water treatment and storage in the home. A practical new strategy to prevent waterborne disease. JAMA. 1995 Mar 22-29;273(12):948-53. http://www.uvm.edu/~bwilcke/reiff.pdf

MENSTRUAL HYGIENE

Why is it necessary?
A comprehensive approach to menstrual hygiene promotion is still a neglected area. The majority of women in the developing world don't have access to sanitary pads, disposal and private washing facilities, which are essential during menstruation. They use rags that are washed quickly (without clean water and soap) and dried in dark places. This is an unhealthy practice, which often leads to infections and illness. Often these infections are left untreated due to shame and ignorance. The problem is not only health, but one of basic human rights and dignity. Sanitary facilities and waste management at schools are often so poor that girls and female teachers prefer not to use these during their menstruation period. This can result in missed classes and prolonged absences.

What is good behaviour?
Girls need to change their menstrual pads regularly during the period of menstruation especially in the first three days. When using rags they should be:
- Soft and clean.
- Washed with soap and dried directly under the sun (to make them germ free) and preferably ironed (against insect eggs).
- Kept in a dry and clean place to use again.
- Should not be shared with others.

If a girl uses pads, she needs to throw them into a pit latrine, bury them, or burn them after use. They should not be flushed down the toilet, as they will cause blockage.

A confidential talk with teachers on how to manage menstrual flow during school days and how to use school facilities would help girls and improve their school attendance. At schools toilets should be available in which girl can change their rags and pads safely, where water is available to wash their hands, and where materials are available to dispose their pads, or in which to wrap their rags.

Example: Sanitary Napkins Machine

Sanitary napkins are now becoming available in remote areas, often using local products for manufacture. Micro-credit programmes can support napkin production as an entrepreneurial activity for women.

Mr A. Muruganantham from Coimbatore in India has designed, tested and implemented a sanitary napkin-making machine that operates on a small scale. Contrary to a large-scale production model this sanitary napkin-making machine can be made available to a buyer for approximately Rs.65,000, (about 1.100 Euro). This allows smaller players to adopt the business model propagated by him, and thus generates more employment in the most neglected sections of society.

The technology used is simple and non-chemical as the machine uses purely mechanical processes such as grinding and defibration, pressing and sealing to convert the raw material – pine wood pulp - into a napkin.

A patent has been obtained for this innovation. Over 125 such machines have been delivered which are now functioning in 14 states of India. Enquiries have come in further afield such as Nigeria, Ethiopia, Kenya Uganda, Nepal and Bangladesh.

Members of the Mahalaxmi Self Help Group in Chhattisgarh State, India, have taken a loan from the bank of Women Self Help Groups to invest in a sanitary napkin-making unit to create a business that employs up to five women. The new invention is capable to make 120 napkins per hour.

(Source: IRC)

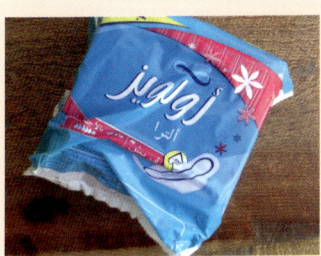 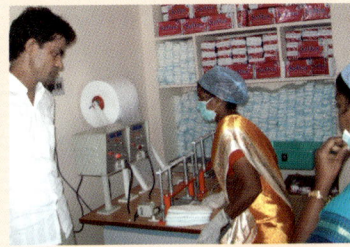

(Source: IRC)

Further Reading
- Download 'India Department of Drinking Water Supply -IN (2008)'. Sharing simple facts useful information about menstrual health and hygiene. New Delhi, India, UNICEF. P27-29 are on menstrual hygiene management in schools.
  http://www.irc.nl/docsearch/title/168685
- Download other information about menstrual hygiene from the IRC website:
  www.irc.nl (search menstrual hygiene).

FOOD PREPARATION & STORAGE

Why is it necessary?
Millions of people fall ill as a result of eating unsafe food, particularly the at-risk groups, such as infants, young children and elderly people. Proper food preparation and storage can prevent many diseases.

Food can be contaminated before it enters the household or within the household due to improper storage, handling or preparation. Some foods such as meat, poultry, vegetables and milk are more likely to become contaminated. Before entering the household, meat and poultry can become contaminated with germs and worms from the animal from which it was taken. It can also become contaminated during processing. Vegetables can become contaminated when irrigated with contaminated water. In the house food can become contaminated when not stored safely, or due to poor hygiene while food is handled and prepared. This can happen when hands are not washed before handling cooked foods, or when contaminated water is used to wash foods that are eaten raw. Therefore preventing stools from getting into the domestic environment and hand washing are priorities for food hygiene as well.

What is good behaviour?
The WHO promotes five key food hygiene messages:
1. Keep clean.
2. Separate raw and cooked food.
3. Cook thoroughly.
4. Keep food at safe temperatures or keep it less than a day.
5. Use safe water and safe raw materials.

Storage options and practices vary greatly between different communities. Many people do not have access to a refrigerator let alone a freezer. Other methods can be used to keep food cool like storing it underground, immersing it in cold water or drying the food. These methods, however, all contain a certain contamination risk. Buying food and slaughtering of animals on a daily basis is usually a safer option.

(Source: PLAN)

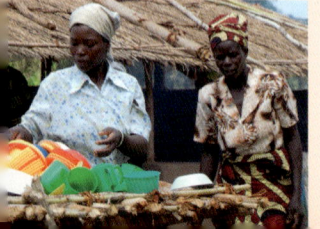

Key lesson 1 "Keep clean"
It is important to keep cooking utensils clean. One way to do so is to let cooking utensils dry on a drying rack after washing them and to store the cooking utensils at a high place, away from the ground. In that way the utensils are less likely to become contaminated. (Source: PLAN)

Case Food Hygiene: The Democratic Republic of Congo
USAID cooperated with the Environmental Health Project and Action Against Hunger-USA in an urban environmental health activity to reduce diarrhoea by improving sanitary conditions in the public markets of Kinshasa. The four key strategies were to: (1) increase the availability of safe drinking water, (2) improve sanitation facilities, (3) establish community management capacity, and (4) improve hygiene practices. Under the project, "sanitation units" (consisting of toilets, showers, water points for washing hands and water storage tanks) were constructed in seven markets, and 11 drinking water points were established in locations where water was not previously available to vendors and customers. Non-governmental organisations and private businesses maintain these new facilities, generating funds by charging fees for their use. Health education specialists use the water points and sanitation units as sites for teaching the market community about hygiene.

The key results of the intervention were:
- Hand washing practices of market restaurateurs and vendors improved noticeably
- Sanitary display of market goods and waste disposal practices improved significantly
- Diarrhoeal disease prevalence among young children of restaurateurs and vendors decreased by 50% (from 25% to 12%).

(Source: EH project USAID)

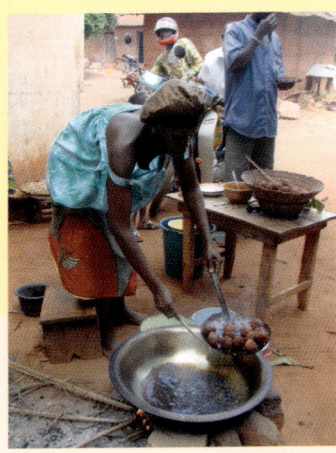

(Source: PLAN)

Further Reading
- Download Food hygiene manual: http://www.who.int/foodsafety/consumer/5keys/en/ http://www.ifh-homehygiene.org/2003/2PUBLIC/ifh_training_resource.pdf
- Download Home hygiene in Developing Countries Prevention of infection in the home and the peri-domestic setting: A training resource on hygiene for teachers, community nurses, community workers and health professionals in developing countries: Sally F. Bloomfield and Kumar J. Nath (WASH & IFH): http://www.ifh-homehygiene.org/2003/2PUBLIC/ifh_training_resource.pdf

Vectors

Vectors may be defined as insects and other animals that are capable of carrying disease causing microorganisms and transmitting these to humans and animals. The presence of vectors is closely linked to hygienic circumstances. If people do not keep their environment and themselves clean, their dwelling will attract insects and animals that may cause or transmit diseases.

Figure 7: Different Vectors.

Vector	Disease Caused (most common)
Mosquitoes	Malaria, Dengue, Yellow Fever, Filariasis and Encephalitis
Non-biting flies	Transmits: Dysentery, Typhoid, Polio and Trachoma
Biting Flies	Sleeping Sickness (TseTse flies), Leishmaniasis (Sand flies) and Onchoserciasis - commonly known as River Blindness- (Black flies)
Rodents	Rabies, Salmonellosis, Lassa Fever and Leptospirosis
Fleas	Plague and Typhus
Lice	Typhus, Relapsing Fever and Skin Infections
Mites	Scabies and other Skin Infections
Ticks	Relapsing Fever, Q-fever
Bedbugs	Anemia
Cockroaches	Transmits: Polio, Amoebas and Intestinal Viruses
Snails	Schistosomiasis -commonly known as bilharzia

(Source: The John Hopkins and IFRC Public Health Guide for Emergencies)

The next two paragraphs will describe tools that can be used to prevent the spread of diseases caused by vectors.

हात धुनै पर्ने अवस्थाहरू

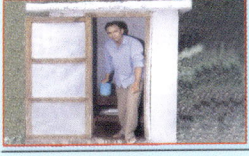
चर्पी प्रयोग गरेपछि
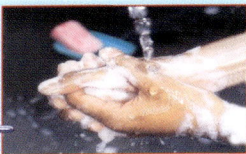

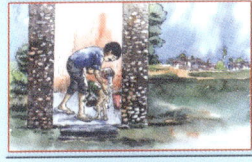
साना नानीको दिसा धोइ दिएपछि
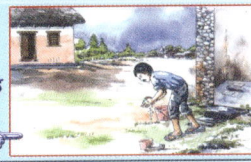

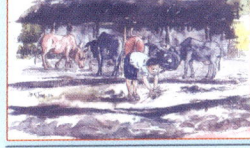
फोहोर छोएपछि
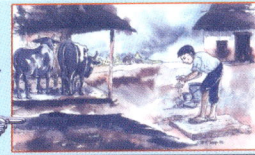

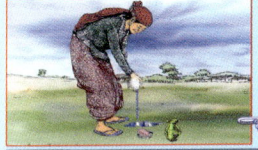
खाना पकाउनु अघि
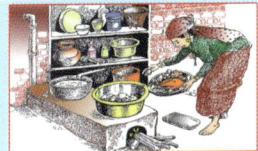

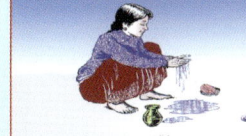
खाना खानु र खुवाउनु अघि
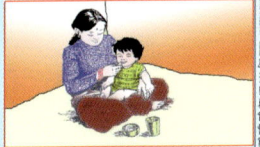

साबुन वा खरानी पानीले राम्ररी हात धोऔं

(Source: IRC)

VECTOR CONTROL

Disposal of waste water and drainage

Why is it necessary?
Water collects in pools, for example from spilling at water points, splashing from bathing, washing clothes and other domestic activities. These pools offer good breeding places for flies and mosquitoes, which may spread diseases. In addition, waste water often contains germs harmful to health. Wastewater should therefore be disposed off carefully. Water points and washing slabs have to be designed in such a way that the waste water is channelled and absorbed into the ground or drained away. Areas where waste water collects need to be kept dry by building drainage and filling holes with earth or sand.

What is good behaviour?
Waste water can be disposed off in several ways:
- It can be used for watering crops if the soil is sufficiently permeable. The water running off from the water point or washing area can then be channelled through (hand dug) sloped trenches lined with plants, which will take out the water from the soils.
- If a septic tank is already built and the size allows it, let the waste water flow into this tank
- Construct a soak pit. In urban areas, a piped drainage system, such as small bore sewerage or regular sewerage may be the best option.

> **Example 1: Drainage at water pump**
> Good drainage is not only important for the disposal of waste water, but is of major importance for limiting the public health hazards of (heavy) rains and floods. If there are areas where rainwater collects regularly then drains can be dug to ensure that these areas stay dry. There are several ways to set up a drainage system, from lined open drains to buried open-jointed pipe drains. Open or closed drains can be used to carry the water to an infiltration field or a soak pit. A silt trap can be installed to remove solids. Drains need to be inspected regularly and rubbish that blocks the drain needs to be removed.

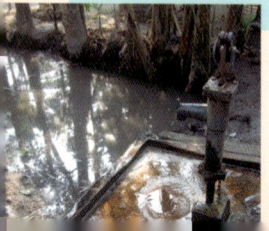
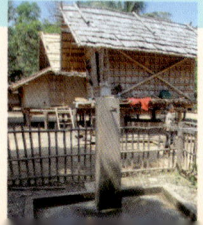

The wrong way and the right way of drainage.

(Source: PLAN)

Example 2: Soak pit

A soak pit, also known as a soak away or leach pit, is a covered, porous-walled chamber that allows water to slowly soak into the ground with or without a piped inlet. The soak pit can be left empty and lined with a porous material, or left unlined and filled with coarse rocks and gravel. The rocks and gravel will prevent the walls from collapsing and prevent breeding, but will still provide adequate space for the waste water. In both cases, a layer of sand and fine gravel should be spread across the bottom to help disperse the flow. The soak pit should be between 1.5 and 4m deep, but never less than 1.5m above the ground water table. Soak pits are best suited to soils with good absorptive properties; clay, hard packed or rocky soils are not appropriate. When the performance of the soak pit deteriorates, the material inside the soak pit can be excavated and refilled (do take hygiene measures into account). To allow for future access, a removable lid should be used to seal the pit until it needs to be maintained.

Figure 8: Soak Pit.

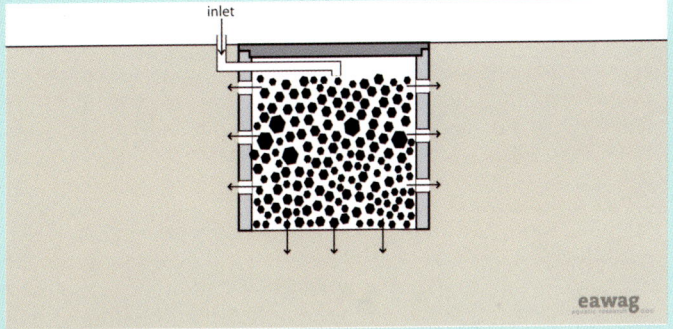

(Source: AKVO)

Further Reading
- Download: Compendium of Sanitation Systems and Technologies (EAWAG): http://www.eawag.ch/organisation/abteilungen/sandec/publikationen/publications_sesp/downloads_sesp/compendium_high.pdf
- Download: Low cost drainage for emergencies. Oxfam Technical Brief. http://www.oxfam.org.uk/resources/downloads/emerg_manuals/draft_oxfam_tech_brief_drainage.pdf
- Website how to build a soak pit: http://www.akvo.org/wiki/index.php/Soak_Pit

VECTOR CONTROL

Solid Waste Disposal

Why is it necessary?
Even though household waste usually does not contain as much germs as excreta, it poses a threat to public health. Waste attracts flies, mosquitoes and rats and offers them a breeding site. The presence of these vectors may spread diseases. In order to prevent vectors from accessing the waste, refuse should always be stored in a container with a tight fitting lid. This container needs to be emptied regularly and be washed with soap or cleaned with dry earth or sand.

What is good behaviour?
If communal refuse collection is not in place, the waste should be divided into 4 groups, which need to be disposed off separately.

1. Vegetable waste, such as leftovers from fruit and vegetables. These can be used for composting, animal food or in some cases in a biogas digester. Do not add remnants of meat or fish to an open compost pile.
2. Plastic bags, containers, tins and glasses can be washed and reused. Problems may arise when these items are not being reused. They do not break down easily and may hold water and subsequently turn into a breeding site for flies and mosquitoes. Therefore these materials should be buried in a covered refuse pit.
3. Letters, newspapers, notebooks, magazines and other paper can be recycled or reused for lighting fires. If paper needs to be thrown away, it can be added to the refuse pit.
4. Dangerous waste such as batteries, used motor oil, kerosene and fuel are hazardous to human health. Care must be taken to prevent this waste from getting into ground water or in other water sources like rivers and streams. This type of waste needs therefore to be put away in a separate pit, which has a sealed base, is covered and is far away from water sources.

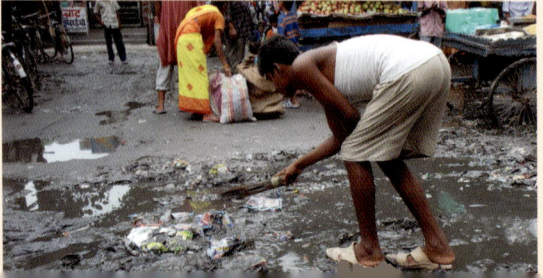

(Source: PLAN)

Example: Refuse Pits

Refuse that cannot be reused can be buried in a pit. When determining the location of this pit the following considerations need to be taken in mind:
- The minimum safe distance from drinking water sources is site specific and should be decided based upon local hydrological and hydro geological conditions.
- The pit needs to be constructed well above the highest likely groundwater level (in the rainy season) in order to prevent contamination of the water supply. If a pit is constructed for hazardous waste, this pit should preferably be situated on impervious rock or clay and have a sealed base.
- The pit should be at least 20 meters away from the food preparation and living area.
- The pit should not be placed above any drainage pipe which discharges into surface water or a drain field.

Further considerations when constructing a refuse pit are:
- The design period of a pit can be increased if the waste is compacted for example by using a wooden pole.
- Children should not be allowed near waste pits.
- Animals need to be kept away from the waste pits.

Further Reading
- Download: Solid Waste Management in Emergencies. WHO Technical Note. http://www.who.int/water_sanitation_health/hygiene/envsan/tn07/en/index.html
- Download: 'Putting Integrated Sustainable Waste Management (ISWM) into practice' http://www.waste.nl/content/search/?SearchText=putting+into+practice&SearchButton=Search
- Download: 'Solid waste management and the Millennium Development Goals' http://www.cwgnet.net/documentation/skatdocumentation.2007-06-28.8568961372/
- Download: Waste Portal (work in progress) http://www.wasteportal.net/ gateway to solid waste management information, focus on low- and middle-income countries

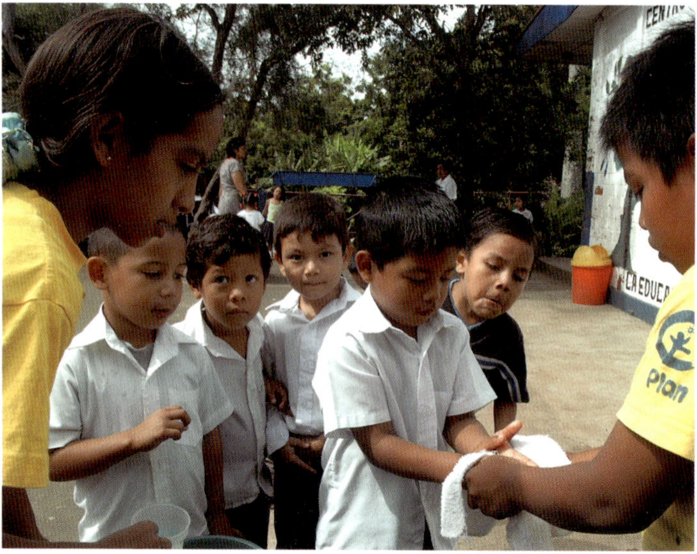

(Source: PLAN)

LITERATURE

Abdallah, S. and Burnham, G.M. (eds) (2004). *The John Hopkins and IFRC Public Health Guide for Emergencies*. Baltimore: LearnWare International Corporation. http://pdf.usaid.gov/pdf_docs/PNACU086.pdf

Almedom et al., (1997). *Hygiene evaluation procedures: approaches and methods for assessing water- and sanitation-related hygiene practices*. International Nutrition Foundation for Developing Countries, Boston. http://www.unu.edu/unupress/food2/UIN11E/UIN11E00.HTM

Curtis, V., et al. (1997) *Dirt and diarrhoea: formative research in hygiene promotion programmes*. Health Policy and Planning: 12(2):122-131, Oxford University Press. http://www.hygienecentral.org.uk/pdf/Formative%20research.pdf

Ensink J. and Curtis V. Well factsheet: *Health impact of hand washing with soap*. http://www.lboro.ac.uk/well/resources/fact-sheets/fact-sheets-htm/Handwashing.htm

IRC (2007). IRC Factsheet: *How to promote measures to prevent water-borne diseases?* http://www.irc.nl/page/8904

IRC (2006). *Children's health clubs in schools. Opportunities and risks*. Developed under the SSHE Global Sharing Project financed by UNICEF. December, 2006.
http://www.schools.watsan.net/redir/content/download/328/2769/file/school%20health%20clubs%20final%20SSHE%20case%20study_WEB.pdf

Jenkins, M. and Sugden, S. (2006). Rethinking Sanitation: *Lessons and innovation for sustainability and success in the new millennium*. Occasional Paper for the Human Development Report 2006 (2006/27). UNDP.
http://hdr.undp.org/en/reports/global/hdr2006/papers/jenkins%20and%20sugden.pdf

Kar, K. & Chambers, R. (2008). *Handbook on Community-Led Total Sanitation*. IDS/Plan, Brighton/London. http://www.communityledtotalsanitation.org/resource/handbook-community-led-total-sanitation

Mintz, E., Reiff, F. & Tauxe, R. (1995). *Safe water treatment and storage in the home*. A practical new strategy to prevent waterborne disease. JAMA. 1995 Mar 22-29;273(12):948-53. http://www.uvm.edu/~bwilcke/reiff.pdf

Peal, A.J. (2010). *Hygiene promotion in South Asia; progress, challenges and emerging issues*. IRC. South Asia hygiene practitioners' workshop. Dhaka, February 2010. http://www.irc.nl/page/51851

UNICEF/WHO (2009). Diarrhoea: *Why children are still dying and what can be done*. United Nations Children's Fund/World Health Organization. New York/Geneva. http://www.unicef.org/health/files/Final_Diarrhoea_Report_October_2009_final.pdf

UNICEF (2008). *UNICEF handbook on water quality*. United Nations Children's Fund, New York.
http://www.unicef.org/wash/files/WQ_Handbook_final_signed_16_April_2008.pdf

Vreede, E. de,(2004). *CHAST in Somalia*. IRC School Sanitation and Hygiene Education Symposium. The way forward: Construction is not enough! Delft, June 2004. http://www.irc.nl/page/13170

WELL (1998). *DFID Guidance manual on water supply and sanitation programmes*. WEDC/Loughborough University, Leicestershire.
http://www.lboro.ac.uk/well/resources/Publications/guidance-manual/guidance-manual.htm

WHO (1997). The PHAST Initiative: *A new approach to working with communities*. World Health Organization, Geneva. Sawyer, R. Simpson, Hebert, M. and Clarke, L.
http://www.who.int/water_sanitation_health/hygiene/envsan/phast/en/

WHO (1998). PHAST Step-by-Step Guide: *a participatory approach for the control of diarrhoeal disease*. World Health Organization, Geneva. Sawyer, R., Simpson – Hebert, M. and Wood, R.
http://www.who.nt/water_sanitation_health/hygiene/envsan/phastep/en/

WHO (2005). State of the world's sight: *VISION 2020: the Right to Sight. 1999-2005*. World Health Organization, Geneva.
http://www.vision2020.org/main.cfm?type=PUBLICATIONS

WSSCC (2009). WSSCC Reference Note: HIV/AIDS and WASH. http://www.wsscc.org/fileadmin/files/pdf/publication/Ref_Note_HIV_AIDS_WASH_February_09.pdf

WSSCC (2010). Hygiene and sanitation software. *An overview of approaches.* Water Supply & Sanitation Collaborative Council, Geneva. Peal, A., Evans, B. and Voorden, C. van der,. http://www.wsscc.org/fileadmin/files/pdf/publication/Hygiene_and_Sanitation_Software_WSSCC_2010.pdf.

3IE (2009). Water, sanitation and hygiene interventions to combat childhood diarrhoea in developing countries International Initiative for Impact Evaluation. *Synthetic Review 001*. Hugh Waddington. Snilstveit, B., White, H. and Fewtrell, L. http://www.3ieimpact.org/page.php?pg=synthetic

References Cases
PHAST: http://www.who.int/water_sanitation_health/hygiene/envsan/en/EOS96-11b.pdf

PHASE: http://www.amref.org/silo/files/phase-program-brochure.pdf

Social Marketing: http://www.irc.nl/page/51637

CLTS: http://www.unicef.org/mozambique/child_survival_5633.html

SLTS: http://www.unicef.org/wash/nepal_39817.html

Community Health Club: http://www.irc.nl/page/38717

School Health Clubs: http://www.webarchive.nationalarchives.gov.uk/+/http://www.dfid.gov.uk/media-room/case-studies/2009/childrens-magazine-makes-healthy-reading-in-indonesia/

References Examples
Tippy Tap: http://www.akvo.org/wiki/index.php?Tippy_Tap

Safe Water Storage: http://www.cawst.org/en/resources/pubs/category/1-cawst-poster-series

Peepoo Bag: http://www.peepoople.com

Sanitary Napkins Machine: http://www.irc.nl/page/51700 & http://www.new-

Food Hygiene: http://www.ehproject.org/PDF/Activity_Reports/AR-19%20%20DRCongoReportFormatted.pdf

Soak Pit: http://www.eawag.ch/organisation/abteilungen/sandec/publikationen/publications_sesp/downloads_sesp/compendium_high.pdf

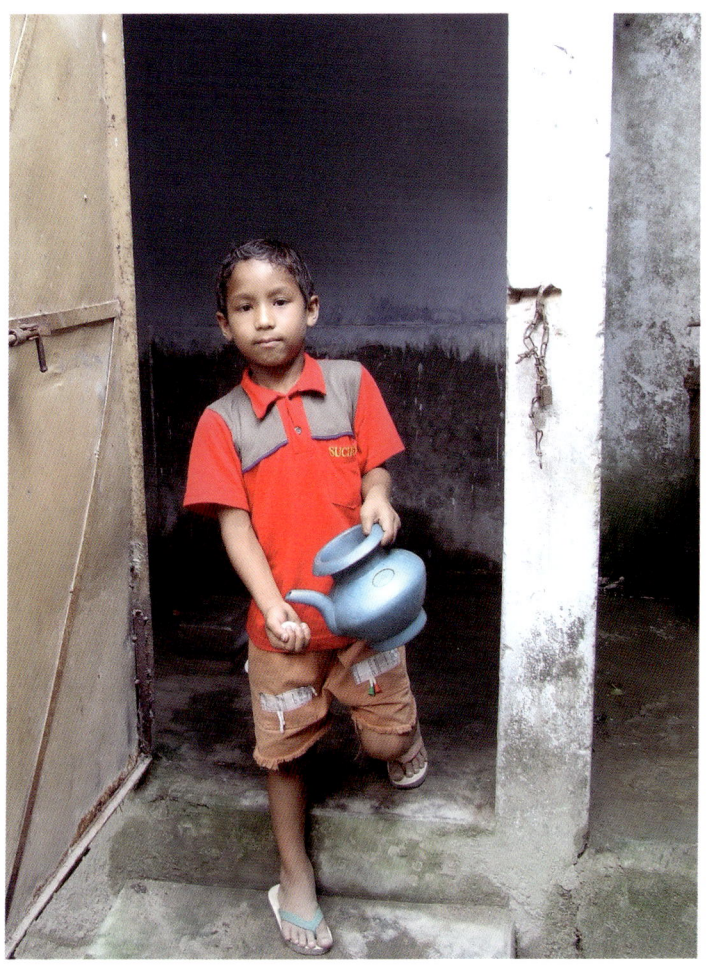

(Source: PLAN)

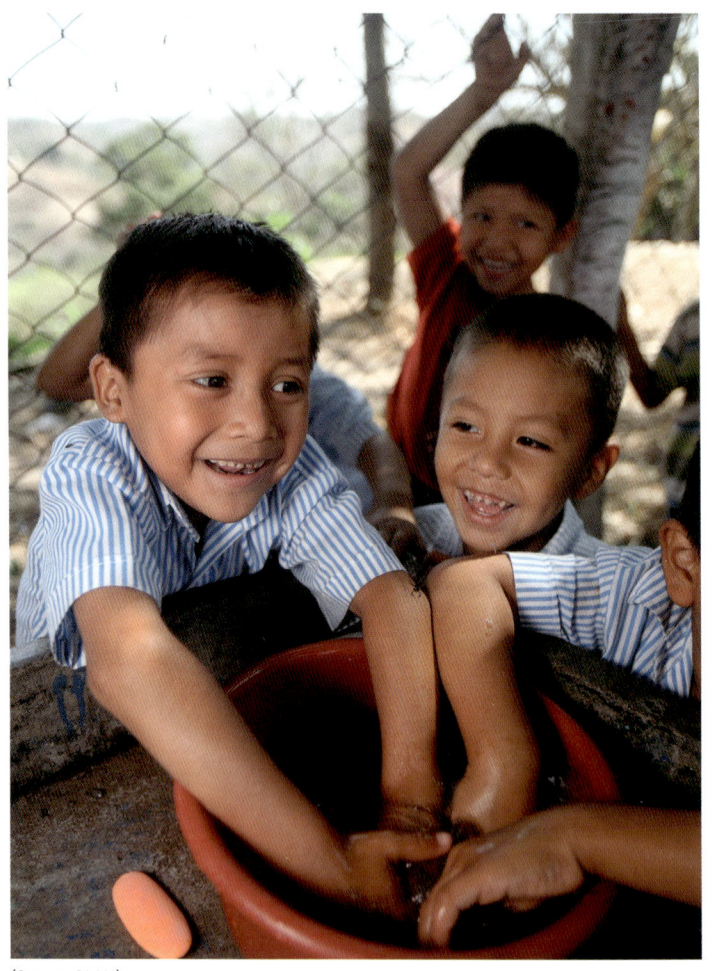

(Source: PLAN)